AUTOIMMUNE HEPATITIS DIET COOKBOOK

Dr. Kimberly Carlos

TABLE OF CONTENT

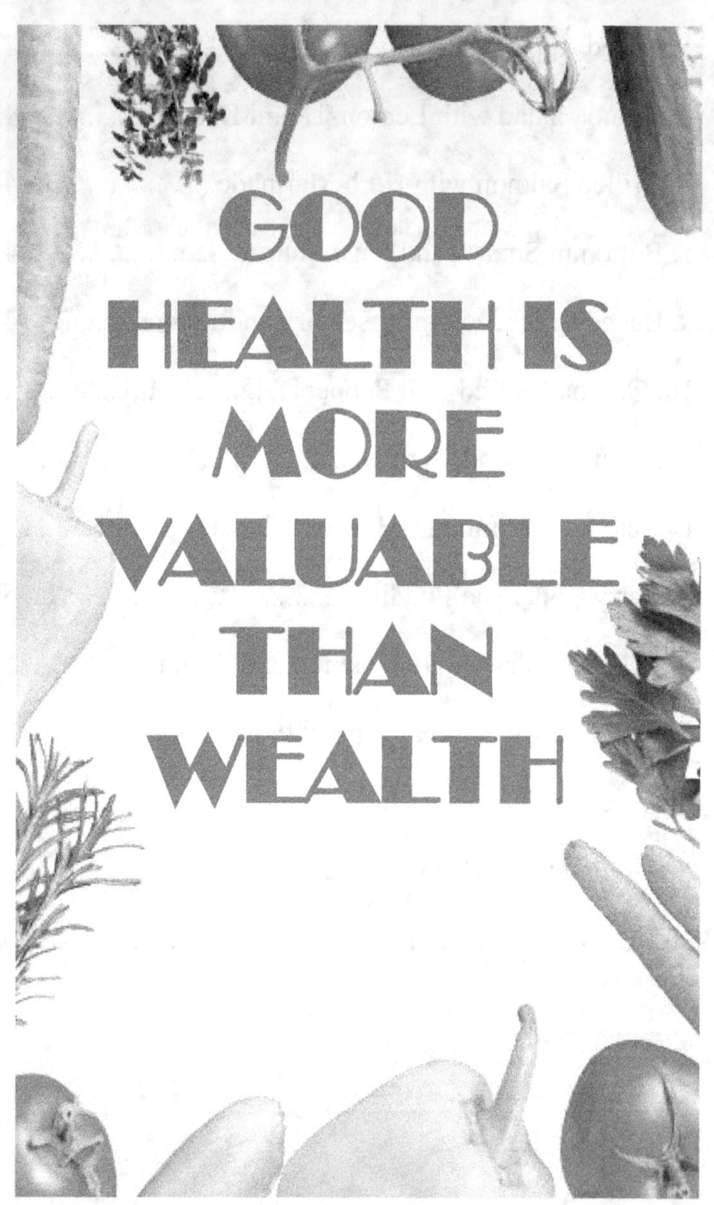
GOOD
HEALTH IS
MORE
VALUABLE
THAN
WEALTH

INTRODUCTION

Welcome to a journey of healing and well-being tailored specifically for those navigating autoimmune hepatitis. In the realm of autoimmune diseases, the liver plays a crucial role, and adopting a thoughtful diet is key to managing symptoms and promoting liver health.

Understanding Autoimmune Hepatitis:

Autoimmune hepatitis is a condition where the body's immune system mistakenly attacks liver cells, leading to inflammation.

Managing this condition involves a holistic approach, and a well-planned diet is a cornerstone of that strategy.

The Power of Nutrition:

A carefully curated diet can significantly impact the course of autoimmune hepatitis. This isn't about restrictive eating; it's about empowering your body with the nutrients it needs to function optimally while minimizing triggers that may exacerbate symptoms.

What to Expect from This Diet Guide:

1. Nutrient-Rich Recipes: Dive into a collection of recipes that prioritize liver-friendly ingredients, aiming to provide the vitamins and minerals necessary for liver function.

2. Dietary Guidelines: Understand the principles of an autoimmune hepatitis-friendly diet. Learn about foods to embrace, those to moderate, and potential triggers to avoid.

3. Balanced and Delicious Meals: Enjoy meals that not only adhere to dietary guidelines but also celebrate flavor and variety. Discover that nourishing your body can be a delightful and satisfying experience.

4. Comprehensive Support: Beyond recipes, this diet guide offers insights into the nutritional aspects of autoimmune hepatitis. It provides information to help you make informed choices about your diet, fostering a sense of control over your well-being.

Why Choose This Diet Guide?

- Tailored for You: Recognizing that each individual's experience with autoimmune hepatitis is unique, this guide offers flexibility and adaptability to suit your specific needs.

- **Holistic Wellness:** Embrace a holistic approach to managing autoimmune hepatitis that encompasses nutrition, self-care, and medical guidance.

- **Flavorful Healing:** Say goodbye to the notion that a therapeutic diet must be bland. These recipes are designed to be delicious, making the healing process enjoyable and sustainable.

Embark on a journey of well-being with the Autoimmune Hepatitis Diet guide. It's more than a collection of recipes; it's a tool to empower you in making choices that contribute to a healthier, more vibrant life. Your liver deserves the best, and this guide is here to support you on your path to wellness.

How to Adopt this Autoimmune Hepatitis Diet Plan

Living with autoimmune hepatitis requires a proactive approach to your health, and a well-thought-out diet plan can be a game-changer.

Here's a step-by-step guide on how to adopt an autoimmune hepatitis diet effectively:

1. Consult Your Healthcare Provider:

- Before making significant changes to your diet, consult with your healthcare provider, especially if you're managing a chronic condition like autoimmune hepatitis.

- Discuss your intention to adopt a specialized diet and seek guidance on how it aligns with your overall treatment plan.

2. Understand the Autoimmune Hepatitis Diet:

- Educate yourself about the autoimmune hepatitis diet. Learn about foods that promote liver health and those that may exacerbate symptoms.

- Understand the principles of a balanced and nutrient-rich diet, emphasizing whole foods and minimizing processed items.

3. Identify Trigger Foods:

- Work with your healthcare provider and a registered dietitian to identify specific trigger foods that may worsen autoimmune hepatitis symptoms.

- Keep a food journal to track your meals and any potential correlations with symptom exacerbation.

4. Embrace Liver-Friendly Foods:

- Prioritize foods that are known to support liver health. This includes a variety of fruits, vegetables, lean proteins, whole grains, and healthy fats.

- Explore recipes that incorporate these liver-friendly ingredients in a way that suits your taste preferences.

5. Gradual Transition:

- Implement changes gradually to allow your body to adapt. Sudden and drastic alterations to your diet may be challenging to sustain.

- Gradual changes also help you monitor how your body responds to specific modifications.

6. Stay Hydrated:

- Adequate hydration is crucial for liver health. Ensure you're drinking enough water throughout the day.

- Limit the consumption of sugary beverages and focus on water, herbal teas, and other hydrating, liver-friendly options.

7. Plan Balanced Meals:

- Plan well-balanced meals that include a mix of macronutrients (carbohydrates, proteins, and fats) and micronutrients (vitamins and minerals).

- Incorporate a rainbow of fruits and vegetables to ensure a diverse range of nutrients.

8. Monitor and Adjust:

- Regularly monitor your symptoms, energy levels, and overall well-being.

- If needed, make adjustments to your diet plan based on your body's responses and consult with your healthcare team for guidance.

Remember, the key is personalized care, and what works for one person may differ for another. Collaborate closely with your healthcare team to tailor an autoimmune hepatitis diet plan that aligns with your health goals and enhances your overall quality of life.

CHAPTER ONE

Delicious Autoimmune Hepatitis Breakfast Recipes

1. Sweet Potato Hash with Spinach and Poached Eggs

Ingredients:

- 1 large sweet potato, peeled and grated

- 1 cup fresh spinach, chopped

- 2 poached eggs

- 1 tablespoon olive oil

- Salt and pepper to taste

- Optional: Fresh herbs for garnish

Instructions:

- Heat olive oil in a skillet over medium heat. Add the grated sweet potato and cook until it starts to brown and becomes tender.

- Stir in the chopped spinach and cook until wilted. Season with salt and pepper to taste.

- While the hash is cooking, poach the eggs in simmering water until the whites are set but the yolks are still runny.

- Plate the sweet potato hash, top with poached eggs, and garnish with fresh herbs if desired. This breakfast is rich in vitamins and provides a good balance of nutrients for individuals with autoimmune hepatitis.

2. Berry and Coconut Chia Pudding Parfait

Ingredients:

- 2 tablespoons chia seeds

- 1/2 cup coconut milk

- 1/2 teaspoon vanilla extract

- 1 cup mixed berries (blueberries, raspberries, strawberries)

- 1 tablespoon shredded coconut

- Optional: Honey or maple syrup for sweetness

Instructions:

- In a bowl, mix chia seeds, coconut milk, and vanilla extract. Stir well and let it sit in the refrigerator for at least 2 hours or overnight until it thickens.

- In a glass or bowl, layer the chia pudding with mixed berries. Repeat the layers, finishing with a sprinkle of shredded coconut on top.

- Drizzle honey or maple syrup over the parfait if you prefer extra sweetness.

- This chia pudding parfait is not only visually appealing but also packed with antioxidants, fiber, and healthy fats.

3. Vegetable Omelette with Herbs

Ingredients:

- 2 eggs

- 1/4 cup diced bell peppers (mixed colors)

- 1/4 cup diced zucchini

- 1/4 cup cherry tomatoes, halved

- 1 tablespoon fresh parsley, chopped

- 1 tablespoon olive oil

- Salt and pepper to taste

Instructions:

- In a bowl, whisk the eggs until well beaten. Season with salt and pepper.

- Heat olive oil in a non-stick skillet over medium heat. Add bell peppers, zucchini, and cherry tomatoes. Sauté until the vegetables are tender.

- Pour the beaten eggs over the sautéed vegetables. Sprinkle fresh parsley on top.

- Allow the eggs to set at the edges. Gently lift the edges with a spatula, letting the uncooked egg flow underneath. Once the omelette is mostly set, fold it in half.

- Slide the vegetable omelette onto a plate. Garnish with additional herbs if desired. This protein-packed breakfast is a delicious way to start the day.

4. Quinoa Breakfast Bowl

Ingredients:

- 1/2 cup cooked quinoa

- 1/4 cup almond milk

- 1/2 banana, sliced

- 1 tablespoon almond butter

- 1 tablespoon chia seeds

- 1 tablespoon chopped walnuts

- Optional: Cinnamon for flavor

Instructions:

- In a bowl, combine cooked quinoa with almond milk. Stir well to combine.

- Top the quinoa mixture with banana slices, almond butter, chia seeds, and chopped walnuts.

- Add a dash of cinnamon for extra flavor.

Enjoy

5. Smoked Salmon Avocado Toast

Ingredients:

- 1 slice whole-grain or gluten-free bread

- 1/2 avocado, mashed

- 2 ounces smoked salmon

- 1 tablespoon capers

- Fresh dill for garnish

- Lemon wedges for serving

Instructions:

- Toast the bread to your liking.

- Spread the mashed avocado evenly over the toasted bread.

- Arrange smoked salmon on top of the avocado.

- Sprinkle capers and garnish with fresh dill.

- Serve the toast with lemon wedges on the side for a burst of citrus flavor.

6. Turmeric Ginger Smoothie

Ingredients:

- 1 cup coconut milk (or any non-dairy milk)

- 1/2 teaspoon turmeric powder

- 1/2 teaspoon grated ginger

- 1/2 cup frozen pineapple chunks

- 1/2 banana

- 1 tablespoon chia seeds

Instructions:

- In a blender, combine coconut milk, turmeric powder, grated ginger, frozen pineapple chunks, banana, and chia seeds.

- Blend until the mixture reaches a smooth consistency.

- Pour the smoothie into a glass and enjoy the anti-inflammatory benefits of turmeric and ginger.

7. Sweet Potato Hash with Poached Eggs

Ingredients:

- 1 medium sweet potato, peeled and grated

- 1 tablespoon olive oil

- 1/2 onion, finely chopped

- 1 garlic clove, minced

- 2 poached eggs

- Salt and pepper to taste

- Fresh parsley for garnish

Instructions:

- In a skillet, heat olive oil over medium heat. Add grated sweet potato, chopped onion, and minced garlic. Cook until sweet potato is tender and slightly crispy.

- Poach two eggs to your liking.

- Place the sweet potato hash on a plate, top with poached eggs, and season with salt and pepper and garnish with fresh parsley for added flavor.

8. Berry and Spinach Smoothie Bowl

Ingredients:

- 1 cup spinach leaves

- 1/2 cup frozen mixed berries (strawberries, blueberries, raspberries)

- 1/2 banana

- 1/2 cup almond milk

- 1 tablespoon almond butter

- Toppings: Fresh berries, sliced banana, granola

Instructions:

- In a blender, combine spinach leaves, frozen berries, banana, almond milk, and almond butter. Blend until smooth.

- Pour the smoothie into a bowl.

- Top with fresh berries, sliced banana, and granola.

Enjoy.

9. Chia Seed Pudding with Berries

Ingredients:

- 2 tablespoons chia seeds

- 1/2 cup unsweetened almond milk

- 1/2 teaspoon vanilla extract

- 1 teaspoon maple syrup (optional)

- Mixed berries for topping

Instructions:

- In a bowl, combine chia seeds, almond milk, vanilla extract, and maple syrup. Stir well.

- Cover the bowl and refrigerate overnight or for at least 4 hours until the chia pudding thickens.

- Once the pudding has set, top it with a variety of mixed berries.

Enjoy

10. Sweet Potato Hash with Spinach and Poached Eggs

Ingredients:

- 1 medium sweet potato, peeled and grated

- 1 cup fresh spinach, chopped

- 2 eggs

- 1 tablespoon olive oil

- Salt and pepper to taste

Instructions:

- In a skillet, heat olive oil over medium heat. Add grated sweet potato and sauté until it becomes golden brown and crispy.

- Add chopped spinach to the sweet potato hash and cook until wilted.

- Meanwhile, poach two eggs to your liking.

- Place the sweet potato hash and spinach on a plate, top with poached eggs, and season with salt and pepper.

Delicious Autoimmune Hepatitis Lunch Recipes

1. Quinoa Salad with Grilled Chicken and Veggies

Ingredients:

- 1 cup quinoa, cooked

- 1 boneless, skinless chicken breast, grilled and sliced

- 1 cup cherry tomatoes, halved

- 1 cucumber, diced

- 1/4 cup red onion, finely chopped

- 2 tablespoons olive oil

- 1 tablespoon balsamic vinegar

- Salt and pepper to taste

- Fresh basil leaves for garnish

Instructions:

- Cook quinoa according to package instructions and let it cool.

- Grill the chicken breast until fully cooked, then slice it into strips.

- In a large bowl, combine the cooked quinoa, grilled chicken, cherry tomatoes, cucumber, and red onion.

- In a small bowl, whisk together olive oil, balsamic vinegar, salt, and pepper.

- Pour the dressing over the salad and toss to combine. Garnish with fresh basil leaves.

- This colorful and protein-packed quinoa salad is a delicious and nutritious lunch option for those following an autoimmune hepatitis diet.

2. Baked Salmon with Roasted Vegetables

Ingredients:

- 2 salmon fillets

- 1 cup broccoli florets

- 1 cup cherry tomatoes, halved

- 1 bell pepper, sliced

- 2 tablespoons olive oil

- 1 teaspoon dried oregano

- 1 teaspoon garlic powder

- Salt and pepper to taste

- Lemon wedges for serving

Instructions:

- Preheat the oven to 400°F (200°C).

- In a baking dish, toss broccoli, cherry tomatoes, and bell pepper with olive oil, dried oregano, garlic powder, salt, and pepper.

- Place the salmon fillets on top of the vegetables. Season the salmon with salt and pepper.

- Bake in the preheated oven for about 15-20 minutes or until the salmon is cooked through and flakes easily with a fork.

- Serve the baked salmon over the roasted vegetables with lemon wedges on the side.

3. Turkey and Vegetable Lettuce Wraps

Ingredients:

- 1 pound ground turkey

- 1 tablespoon olive oil

- 1 onion, finely chopped

- 2 cloves garlic, minced

- 1 zucchini, grated

- 1 carrot, grated

- 1 teaspoon ground cumin

- 1 teaspoon paprika

- Salt and pepper to taste

- Iceberg lettuce leaves for wrapping

Instructions:

- In a skillet, heat olive oil over medium heat. Add ground turkey and cook until browned.

- Add chopped onion, minced garlic, grated zucchini, and grated carrot to the skillet. Cook until vegetables are tender.

- Season the mixture with ground cumin, paprika, salt, and pepper. Stir well to combine.

- Spoon the turkey and vegetable mixture onto individual iceberg lettuce leaves.

- These flavorful and low-carb lettuce wraps make a satisfying and autoimmune hepatitis-friendly lunch option.

4. Sweet Potato and Kale Hash with Poached Eggs

Ingredients:

- 2 sweet potatoes, peeled and diced

- 2 cups kale, chopped

- 1 tablespoon coconut oil

- 1 teaspoon smoked paprika

- Salt and pepper to taste

- 4 eggs, poached

Instructions:

- Preheat the oven to 400°F (200°C). Toss diced sweet potatoes with coconut oil, smoked paprika, salt, and pepper. Roast until golden and tender.

- In a skillet, sauté chopped kale until wilted.

- Mix the roasted sweet potatoes with sautéed kale. Poach eggs and place them on top of the sweet potato and kale hash.

- Enjoy this nutrient-rich and hearty hash as a delicious autoimmune hepatitis-friendly lunch.

5. Mediterranean Chickpea Salad

Ingredients:

- 1 can (15 oz) chickpeas, drained and rinsed

- 1 cucumber, diced

- 1 cup cherry tomatoes, halved

- 1/2 red onion, finely chopped

- 1/4 cup Kalamata olives, sliced

- 1/4 cup feta cheese, crumbled

- 2 tablespoons olive oil

- 1 tablespoon red wine vinegar

- 1 teaspoon dried oregano

- Salt and pepper to taste

Instructions:

- In a large bowl, combine chickpeas, diced cucumber, cherry tomatoes, chopped red onion, sliced Kalamata olives, and crumbled feta cheese.

- In a small bowl, whisk together olive oil, red wine vinegar, dried oregano, salt, and pepper.

- Pour the dressing over the salad and toss gently to combine.

6. Grilled Salmon with Lemon and Dill

Ingredients:

- 4 salmon fillets

- 2 tablespoons fresh dill, chopped

- 1 lemon, sliced

- Salt and pepper to taste

- Olive oil for grilling

Instructions:

- Preheat your grill to medium-high heat.

- Season salmon fillets with salt, pepper, and chopped fresh dill.

- Place the salmon fillets on the preheated grill. Grill each side for about 4-5 minutes or until the salmon is cooked through and has a nice grill mark.

- Garnish with lemon slices and serve this delicious grilled salmon as a nutritious and flavorful dinner option.

7. Quinoa and Vegetable Stir-Fry

Ingredients:

- 1 cup quinoa, cooked

- 1 cup broccoli florets

- 1 bell pepper, sliced

- 1 carrot, julienned

- 1 cup snap peas

- 2 tablespoons soy sauce (gluten-free)

- 1 tablespoon sesame oil

- 1 teaspoon ginger, minced

- 2 cloves garlic, minced

- Green onions for garnish

Instructions:

- Cook quinoa according to package instructions and set aside.

- In a large wok or skillet, heat sesame oil. Add ginger and garlic, then stir in broccoli, bell pepper, carrot, and snap peas. Stir-fry until vegetables are tender-crisp.

- Add cooked quinoa to the stir-fried vegetables. Pour soy sauce over the mixture and toss to combine.

- Garnish with green onions and serve this nutrient-packed quinoa and vegetable stir-fry for a satisfying and autoimmune hepatitis-friendly dinner.

8. Baked Chicken with Rosemary and Garlic

Ingredients:

- 4 boneless, skinless chicken breasts

- 2 tablespoons olive oil

- 3 cloves garlic, minced

- 1 tablespoon fresh rosemary, chopped

- Salt and pepper to taste

- Lemon wedges for serving

Instructions:

- Preheat your oven to 400°F (200°C).

- Place chicken breasts in a baking dish. Drizzle with olive oil and rub minced garlic, chopped rosemary, salt, and pepper over the chicken.

- Bake in the preheated oven for 25-30 minutes or until the chicken is cooked through and juices run clear.

- Squeeze lemon wedges over the baked chicken before serving. This flavorful and simple baked chicken is a delightful addition to your autoimmune hepatitis-friendly dinner options.

9. Zucchini Noodles with Pesto Sauce

Ingredients:

- 4 medium-sized zucchinis, spiralized

- 1 cup cherry tomatoes, halved

- 1/2 cup pine nuts, toasted

- 1/2 cup fresh basil leaves

- 1/4 cup nutritional yeast

- 2 cloves garlic

- 1/2 cup olive oil

- Salt and pepper to taste

Instructions:

- Spiralize the zucchinis to create zucchini noodles.

- In a blender, combine fresh basil, pine nuts, nutritional yeast, garlic, olive oil, salt, and pepper. Blend until smooth.

- Toss the zucchini noodles and cherry tomatoes with the pesto sauce until well coated.

- Enjoy this light and flavorful zucchini noodle dish as a delicious and autoimmune hepatitis-friendly dinner.

10. Eggplant and Chickpea Curry

Ingredients:

- 1 large eggplant, diced

- 1 can (15 oz) chickpeas, drained and rinsed

- 1 onion, finely chopped

- 3 tomatoes, chopped

- 3 cloves garlic, minced

- 1 tablespoon curry powder

- 1 teaspoon ground cumin

- 1 teaspoon ground coriander

- 1/2 teaspoon turmeric

- 1 can (14 oz) coconut milk

- Salt and pepper to taste

- Fresh cilantro for garnish

Instructions:

- In a large pot, sauté chopped onion and minced garlic until softened. Add diced eggplant and cook until lightly browned.

- Stir in curry powder, ground cumin, ground coriander, and turmeric. Cook for 1-2 minutes until fragrant.

- Add chopped tomatoes, chickpeas, and coconut milk. Season with salt and pepper. Simmer until the eggplant is tender.

Delicious Autoimmune Hepatitis Breakfast Dinner Recipes

1. Quinoa Breakfast Bowl

Ingredients:

- 1 cup quinoa, cooked

- 1 cup mixed berries (blueberries, strawberries, raspberries)

- 1 tablespoon chia seeds

- 1 tablespoon hemp seeds

- 1 tablespoon almond butter

- 1 teaspoon honey or maple syrup

- A handful of chopped nuts (walnuts, almonds, or pecans)

- Fresh mint leaves for garnish

Instructions:

- In a bowl, combine cooked quinoa, mixed berries, chia seeds, and hemp seeds.

- Drizzle almond butter over the quinoa and berry mixture.

- Add honey or maple syrup for sweetness. Top with chopped nuts and garnish with fresh mint leaves.

- Enjoy this nutrient-packed quinoa breakfast bowl, providing essential vitamins and antioxidants.

2. Avocado Toast with Smoked Salmon

Ingredients:

- 2 slices gluten-free bread, toasted

- 1 ripe avocado

- Juice of 1 lemon

- Salt and pepper to taste

- 4 oz smoked salmon

- Fresh dill for garnish

Instructions:

- Mash the ripe avocado in a bowl and mix it with lemon juice, salt, and pepper.

- Toast the gluten-free bread slices until golden brown.

- Spread the mashed avocado evenly over the toasted bread slices.

- Arrange smoked salmon on top of the avocado-covered toast.

- Garnish with fresh dill and serve this delightful avocado toast with smoked salmon for a delicious and nutritious breakfast.

3. Sweet Potato and Spinach Hash

Ingredients:

- 2 medium sweet potatoes, peeled and grated

- 2 cups fresh spinach, chopped

- 1 onion, finely chopped

- 2 cloves garlic, minced

- 1 teaspoon cumin powder

- Salt and pepper to taste

- 2 tablespoons olive oil

- Poached eggs for serving (optional)

Instructions:

- In a large skillet, heat olive oil over medium heat. Add chopped onions and minced garlic. Sauté until softened.

- Add grated sweet potatoes to the skillet. Cook until they start to brown and become crispy.

- Stir in chopped spinach, cumin powder, salt, and pepper. Cook until spinach wilts.

- Optionally, serve the hash with poached eggs on top for a protein boost. Enjoy this nutrient-rich and flavorful breakfast.

4. Turmeric Smoothie Bowl

Ingredients:

- 1 frozen banana

- 1 cup frozen mango chunks

- 1 cup coconut milk

- 1 teaspoon turmeric powder

- 1/2 teaspoon ginger, grated

- Toppings: Chia seeds, shredded coconut, sliced almonds, fresh berries

Instructions:

- In a blender, combine frozen banana, frozen mango, coconut milk, turmeric powder, and grated ginger. Blend until smooth.

- Pour the smoothie into a bowl and level the surface.

- Sprinkle chia seeds, shredded coconut, sliced almonds, and fresh berries on top.

- Dive into this vibrant turmeric smoothie bowl, packed with anti-inflammatory properties and delicious flavors.

5. Baked Apple Oatmeal Cups

Ingredients:

- 2 cups rolled oats

- 1 teaspoon baking powder

- 1 teaspoon cinnamon

- 1/4 teaspoon salt

- 1 1/2 cups almond milk

- 1/4 cup maple syrup

- 2 apples, diced

- 1/3 cup chopped nuts (walnuts or almonds)

- Coconut oil (for greasing muffin tin)

Instructions:

- Preheat the oven to 350°F (175°C). Grease a muffin tin with coconut oil.

- In a bowl, combine rolled oats, baking powder, cinnamon, and salt.

- Stir in almond milk and maple syrup. Mix well.

- Gently fold in diced apples and chopped nuts.

- Spoon the mixture into the muffin tin. Bake for 25-30 minutes or until the tops are golden brown.

- Allow the oatmeal cups to cool before serving. These baked apple oatmeal cups make a delightful and nutritious breakfast option.

6. Quinoa Salad with Lemon-Tahini Dressing

Ingredients:

- 1 cup cooked quinoa

- 1 cup cucumber, diced

- 1 cup cherry tomatoes, halved

- 1/2 cup red bell pepper, chopped

- 1/4 cup red onion, finely chopped

- 1/4 cup fresh parsley, chopped

- 2 tablespoons olive oil

- 2 tablespoons tahini

- Juice of 1 lemon

- Salt and pepper to taste

Instructions:

- Cook quinoa according to package instructions and let it cool.

- In a large bowl, combine cooked quinoa, cucumber, cherry

tomatoes, red bell pepper, red onion, and fresh parsley.

- In a small bowl, whisk together olive oil, tahini, lemon juice, salt, and pepper.

- Drizzle the lemon-tahini dressing over the salad and toss to coat evenly.

- Serve this refreshing quinoa salad as a light lunch or side dish.

7. Grilled Salmon with Herb Marinade

Ingredients:

- 2 salmon fillets

- 2 tablespoons olive oil

- 1 tablespoon fresh dill, chopped

- 1 tablespoon fresh parsley, chopped

- 1 clove garlic, minced

- Zest of 1 lemon

- Salt and pepper to taste

Instructions:

- Preheat the grill to medium-high heat.

- In a bowl, mix olive oil, chopped dill, chopped parsley, minced garlic, lemon zest, salt, and pepper.

- Coat the salmon fillets with the herb marinade, ensuring they are well-covered.

- Grill the salmon for 4-5 minutes per side or until it flakes easily with a fork.

- Plate the grilled salmon and garnish with additional herbs. Enjoy this protein-rich dish that's gentle on the liver.

8. Butternut Squash and Sage Soup

Ingredients:

- 1 medium butternut squash, peeled and cubed

- 1 onion, chopped

- 2 carrots, chopped

- 2 celery stalks, chopped

- 4 cups vegetable broth

- 2 tablespoons olive oil

- 1 tablespoon fresh sage, chopped

- Salt and pepper to taste

- Coconut milk (optional, for garnish)

Instructions:

- In a large pot, heat olive oil and sauté chopped onion, carrots, and celery until softened.

- Add butternut squash cubes and chopped sage to the pot. Stir well.

- Pour vegetable broth into the pot. Bring to a boil, then reduce heat and simmer until the vegetables are tender.

- Use an immersion blender to puree the soup until smooth. Season with salt and pepper.

- Ladle the butternut squash and sage soup into bowls. Optionally, drizzle with coconut milk for added richness.

9. Baked Chicken with Rosemary and Lemon

Ingredients:

- 2 boneless, skinless chicken breasts

- 2 tablespoons olive oil

- 1 tablespoon fresh rosemary, chopped

- Zest and juice of 1 lemon

- Salt and pepper to taste

Instructions:

- Preheat the oven to 375°F (190°C).

- In a bowl, mix olive oil, chopped rosemary, lemon zest, lemon juice, salt, and pepper.

- Coat the chicken breasts with the marinade, ensuring they are well-covered.

- Place the marinated chicken breasts on a baking sheet and bake for 25-30 minutes or until cooked through.

- Slice the baked chicken and serve it with a side of steamed vegetables for a wholesome meal.

10. Quinoa-Stuffed Bell Peppers

Ingredients:

- 4 bell peppers, halved and seeds removed

- 1 cup cooked quinoa

- 1 can black beans, drained and rinsed

- 1 cup corn kernels

- 1 cup cherry tomatoes, diced

- 1/2 cup fresh cilantro, chopped

- 1 teaspoon ground cumin

- 1 teaspoon chili powder

- Salt and pepper to taste

- 1 cup shredded lettuce (for garnish)

Instructions:

- Preheat the oven to 375°F (190°C). Place the halved bell peppers on a baking sheet.

- In a bowl, combine cooked quinoa, black beans, corn,

cherry tomatoes, cilantro, cumin, chili powder, salt, and pepper.

- Spoon the quinoa mixture into each bell pepper half.

- Bake for 20-25 minutes or until the peppers are tender.

- Garnish with shredded lettuce and serve these quinoa-stuffed bell peppers as a colorful and nutritious dish.

11. Mango Avocado Salsa

Ingredients:

- 1 ripe mango, diced

- 1 avocado, diced

- 1/2 red onion, finely chopped

- 1 jalapeño, seeds removed and finely chopped

- Juice of 2 limes

- 2 tablespoons fresh cilantro, chopped

- Salt and pepper to taste

Instructions:

- In a bowl, combine diced mango, diced avocado, chopped red onion, chopped jalapeño, lime juice, cilantro, salt, and pepper.

- Gently toss all the ingredients until well combined.

- Allow the salsa to chill in the refrigerator for at least 30 minutes to let the flavors meld.

- Serve the refreshing mango avocado salsa with grilled chicken or fish for a light and flavorful accompaniment.

Delicious Autoimmune Hepatitis Dessert Recipes

1. Berry Chia Seed Pudding

Ingredients:

- 1/4 cup chia seeds

- 1 cup unsweetened almond milk

- 1 teaspoon pure vanilla extract

- 1 tablespoon maple syrup (optional)

- Mixed berries for topping

Instructions:

1. In a bowl, combine chia seeds, almond milk, vanilla extract, and maple syrup.

2. Stir well and let it sit in the refrigerator for at least 2 hours or overnight until it thickens.

3. Top with a variety of mixed berries before serving.

2. Baked Apples with Cinnamon and Walnuts

Ingredients:

- 2 apples, cored and halved

- 2 tablespoons chopped walnuts

- 1 teaspoon ground cinnamon

- 1 tablespoon melted coconut oil

- 1 tablespoon honey (optional)

Instructions:

1. Preheat the oven to 375°F (190°C).

2. Place apple halves in a baking dish.

3. In a small bowl, mix chopped walnuts, cinnamon, melted coconut oil, and honey.

4. Spoon the mixture onto each apple half.

5. Bake for 25-30 minutes or until apples are tender.

3. Coconut Milk Panna Cotta with Berries

Ingredients:

- 1 can (13.5 oz) full-fat coconut milk

- 2 tablespoons honey or maple syrup

- 1 teaspoon vanilla extract

- 1 tablespoon grass-fed gelatin

- Mixed berries for topping

Instructions:

1. In a saucepan, heat coconut milk over low heat.

2. Whisk in honey (or maple syrup) and vanilla extract until well combined.

3. Sprinkle gelatin over the mixture and whisk continuously until the gelatin dissolves.

4. Pour the mixture into individual molds or ramekins and refrigerate for at least 4 hours or until set.

5. Top with mixed berries before serving.

4. Avocado Chocolate Mousse

Ingredients:

- 2 ripe avocados

- 1/4 cup unsweetened cocoa powder

- 1/4 cup honey or maple syrup

- 1 teaspoon vanilla extract

- Pinch of sea salt

Instructions:

1. In a blender or food processor, combine avocados, cocoa powder, honey (or maple syrup), vanilla extract, and a pinch of sea salt.

2. Blend until smooth and creamy.

3. Refrigerate for at least 1 hour before serving.

5. Almond Flour Banana Bread

Ingredients:

- 2 cups almond flour

- 1 teaspoon baking soda

- 1/2 teaspoon salt

- 3 ripe bananas, mashed

- 3 large eggs

- 1/4 cup coconut oil, melted

- 1 teaspoon vanilla extract

- 1/2 cup chopped nuts (optional)

Instructions:

1. Preheat the oven to 350°F (175°C) and grease a loaf pan.

2. In a bowl, whisk together almond flour, baking soda, and salt.

3. In another bowl, combine mashed bananas, eggs, melted coconut oil, and vanilla extract.

4. Add the wet ingredients to the dry ingredients and stir until well combined.

5. Fold in chopped nuts if desired.

6. Pour the batter into the loaf pan and bake for 50-60 minutes or until a toothpick comes out clean.

CONCLUSION

In conclusion, this Autoimmune Hepatitis Diet Cookbook serves as a comprehensive guide to navigating a dietary path that not only supports overall health but is specifically tailored to individuals managing Autoimmune Hepatitis.

Through an array of delicious recipes, carefully crafted with ingredients mindful of liver health and autoimmune conditions, this cookbook aims to make the journey towards a balanced and enjoyable diet more accessible.

Each recipe is a testament to the belief that managing health conditions doesn't mean sacrificing flavor or variety. By incorporating nutrient-dense and liver-friendly ingredients, these recipes provide a satisfying culinary experience while adhering to the dietary considerations necessary for those with Autoimmune Hepatitis.

This cookbook is not just a collection of recipes; it's a tool for empowerment, offering individuals the means to take charge of their well-being through mindful and enjoyable eating. As the final page turns, it is our hope that this cookbook becomes a trusted companion in the kitchen, inspiring a journey towards health, balance, and the joy of delicious, nourishing meals tailored to the unique needs of those with Autoimmune Hepatitis.

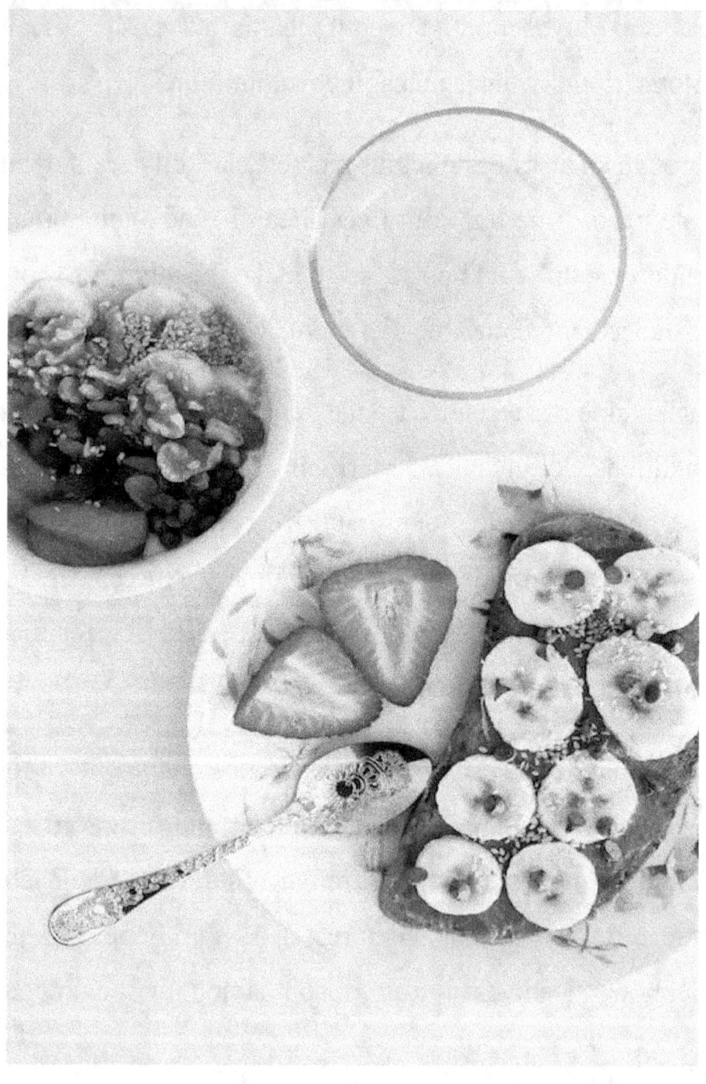